Raquel Elizabeth Rivera Vargas
Karen Pamela Llerena Quishpe
Salvador Alberola Enguix

Physiotherapeutic intervention from Person-Centered Care

Raquel Elizabeth Rivera Vargas
Karen Pamela Llerena Quishpe
Salvador Alberola Enguix

Physiotherapeutic intervention from Person-Centered Care

Proposal for physiotherapeutic intervention in the elderly

ScienciaScripts

Imprint

Cover image: www.ingimage.com

This book is a translation from the original published under ISBN 978-620-0-02104-5.

Publisher:
Sciencia Scripts
is a trademark of
Dodo Books Indian Ocean Ltd. and OmniScriptum S.R.L publishing group

120 High Road, East Finchley, London, N2 9ED, United Kingdom
Str. Armeneasca 28/1, office 1, Chisinau MD-2012, Republic of Moldova, Europe
Managing Directors: Ieva Konstantinova, Victoria Ursu
info@omniscriptum.com

Printed at: see last page
ISBN: 978-620-8-60942-9

Proposal for physiotherapeutic intervention from the perspective of Person-Centred Care.

AUTHORS:

Rivera Vargas, Raquel Elizabeth

Karen Pamela Llerena Quishpe

Salvador Alberola Enguix

Content

1. Summary

This proposal for physiotherapeutic intervention is based on the Person-Centred Care Model, which encompasses two important points: the first point is physiotherapeutic treatment to improve the quality of life and skills when carrying out the activities of daily living of each user, and the second is to investigate the life history in order to have a comprehensive approach to the older adult. The period of application was short due to the situation of confinement due to the pandemic. Nevertheless, it was possible to observe in the residents an improvement in muscular strength, coordination when carrying out activities and a better predisposition to carry out the exercises, with an adequate state of mind.

The experience in the application also generated changes in the therapist-patient dialogue, it was modified to a dialogue of fellow residents, the hierarchy is maintained, it is a horizontal treatment, the user intervenes in the treatment planning. As a health professional, the vision of work was modified, as I learned important details of people's lives, hobbies, sports and activities that I used to do in other stages of my life. Therapy was approached with a different, assertive and holistic approach. Considering that the residents are older adults with dementia or depression problems, the application of individualised therapy did not give rise to difficulties in carrying out the exercise, in one resident the exercise scheme was modified due to states of anxiety .

A second objective in the intervention proposal was to create a Physiotherapy Medical Record based on the Person-Centred Care Model. To this end, information was collected in two ways: the first was information from the interdisciplinary team of the Residence and the second was unstructured interviews with residents and carers. The information collected was captured in a Person-Centred Comprehensive Physiotherapy Medical Record.

A third objective was to capture the Life History of the resident in the global Clinical History of the Residence, the information was obtained in conversations with the users, family and carers, although time was limited, the Life History was elaborated and filed in the Logbook of each resident.

For best results, it is recommended to apply the therapeutic treatment for 2 months .

Keywords: older adult, geriatric centres, person-centred care, physiotherapy, life history, clinical history, interview

2. Introduction and justification

In a globalised world, where life expectancy has increased, the World Health Organisation (WHO, 2017) reports that by 2050 the number of people over 60 years of age will double, which is why it is important to give greater focus to the Geriatric Health Area, creating intervention programmes for the support and care of older adults. Considering the directly proportional relationship between the increase in life expectancy and comorbidities, psychological, social and family problems, it is necessary to create interdisciplinary teams and intervention programmes for the treatment and care of the elderly.

According to the geriatric problems that a person may have, the attention of the interdisciplinary team is required, with the mission of providing the person with quality and warmth care. Physiotherapy is part of this team, and its fundamental objective is to maintain the person's greater independence in their environment and in their activities of daily living. The Person-Centred Care Model (MACP) helps us to have a more humane, individual, empathic vision, a better doctor-patient relationship and a better interdisciplinary team. The older adult is considered as a person capable of making decisions despite their health problems (Díaz et al., 2017). In the MACP, information about the family environment, preferences and hobbies are considered in order to provide a humane and appropriate treatment to the older adult. Considering the benefits of MACP, it is important to modify the physiotherapist's vision in order to have a better response to the treatment of residents.

In daily practice, the therapist focuses on treatments and protocols to be followed for a specific purpose, without giving more relevance to the person. The present intervention proposal is to design and apply a physiotherapeutic intervention based on the principles of Person-Centred Care (PCA). The proposed intervention is aimed at people with dementia and problems of coordination and balance. With the help of the interdisciplinary team, the clinical history is analysed and information collected through interviews with the residents and their relatives is analysed in order to elaborate their life history; their preferences are also asked about, for example, the music to be used in the therapeutic sessions in order to personalise them.

3. Theoretical framework

3.1. Person-Centred Care

Focused on providing a better quality of life for the elderly, physiotherapy from the perspective of the MACP and the support of the interdisciplinary team, the treatment perspective is modified to focus on an optimal, participatory, individual therapy based on the biopsychosocial needs of the person.

According to WHO (1994), quality of life is an individual's perception of his or her place in existence, in the context of the culture and value system in which he or she lives and in relation to his or her goals, expectations, norms and concerns. Health-related quality of life is the ability of the individual to perform those important activities related to the functional, affective and social component, influenced by subjective perception. The ageing process generates important changes in the lifestyle of the population and has significant repercussions on the volume and distribution of the social burden of disease and on quality of life (Botero and Pico, 2007). Based on improving the quality of life, there are changes in the models of care for older adults, the older adult is considered as the axis to participate in decisions about their health and care.

Person-centred therapy is the guideline for the beginnings of PCA, it is based on a humanistic approach, the person is the central focus. It is characterised by the development of the person as a dignified interdependent individual and his or her relationship to the environment. It is based on enhancing individual, social and psychological characteristics, generating decision-making strategies, improving creativity and self-fulfilment of the older adult (Martínez, 2013).

The main focus of the MACP is the user, its aim is to improve their quality of life while maintaining their autonomy and well-being. In order to train organisations, institutions and professionals in the application of this model of care, principles, statements and foundations have been developed, generating an internal organisation and a change in the approach to user care.

For Yanguas and Rabadán (2017) the model of care for the person places the elderly person as an active agent offering care that recognises the person regardless of their status as a unique being and their right to decide on their care and daily life, the components that stand out in this model are

- The person is the fundamental axis; the individual is considered unique, autonomous, with the power to decide on his or her well-being, care, activities, residence, assets.
- Being the protagonist in decision making, he/she plans with the interdisciplinary team activities according to his/her experiences, experiences and tastes, creating a pleasant routine, with meaningful activities and a homely atmosphere.
- The emotional ties created in a person's life are fundamental and it is important that the person maintains a good social relationship with his or her family and friends.
- The physical space is one of the important points in the MACP, to be a homely environment, allowing the elderly to stay in a warm and welcoming place and not a hospital ward, for this reason the residences have a homely aspect. The room is the personalised space of the elderly, in this space the most significant objects of each resident will be located, it is the safe with elements that tell their life, their history, their essence as a person, their memories.

The principles of ACP are based on comprehensiveness and personalisation. Comprehensiveness is treating the person as unique, important, individual and autonomous, respecting the decisions and wishes about their care. Personalisation means considering that the person has the right to live in a home-like setting, with space to place his or her life memories and most precious belongings, and has the right to be surrounded by professionals who treat him or her as family. The principles outlined by ethics in relation to clinical care practice in which ACP is developed (Díaz et al., 2017) are:

- Non-maleficence, the most important principle, is based on providing our service to the person, without intending to harm him or her, to damage his or her integrity and not to trample on his or her dignity as an individual.
- Justice, every person has the right not to be discriminated against under any circumstances, their race, creed, culture, thought must be respected, as health personnel we are obliged to prevent, intervene and follow up on problems related to mistreatment or discrimination.
- Autonomy, every individual is unique, indivisible and irreplaceable, to be respected and valued, without discrimination to his or her moral code, values and beliefs.
- Beneficence, every elderly person has the right to have a good quality of life, with optimal care in any field and to be treated with respect and understanding.

For Martínez (2013) the foundations of PCA are: the person as the central axis, self-determination, ethics, regulations and scientific knowledge . The person is considered as an independent autonomous being who should be treated with respect, tolerance, dignity and based on the strict principles of bioethics. In order to establish the schedule of activities for the care of the elderly, the professionals consider the preferences, hobbies and activities that are not to the user's liking.

The ACP is based on and aligned with the main statements and recommendations of various international standards and consensus. It is guided and informed by scientific knowledge, integrating people's preferences and respect for them with evidence-based interventions that have demonstrated therapeutic benefit for older people.

The basic rules or decalogue for the application of PCA (Díaz-Veiga et al., 2017) are:

All people are dynamic multidimensional beings, who should be treated with dignity, considered as unique beings, the life story is the essential part of the user, the biography, experiences, capabilities, skills, strengths, joys, sorrows, relationships, family, friends, challenges and projects in different stages are told; the person is visualised as an autonomous being with the right to take decisions about their health, residence, food and related situations that affect their life, despite having a cognitive impairment.

The home or residence should have guidelines for the user to feel comfortable during their stay, this should be a homely, warm, welcoming, familiar environment. A relaxed environment, with adequate lighting, comfortable, the environment will influence behaviour and subjective wellbeing; the user living in a residence can have access to carry out daily activities that are important and significant. Keeping the family and friends bond active generates tranquillity, a sense of well-being and emotional stability in the person (Díaz et al., 2017).

The study by Howard et al, (2016), indicates that the goal of the health care leader is to provide a comprehensive and holistic approach to improving the lives of older adults; it reports that with the right resources and support, older adults can actualise their potential to become their own "health care leader", take responsibility for their wellbeing and pursue their self-identified personal goals.

The proposed multifactorial person-centred nursing intervention developed by Ha and Park (2020) was an intervention to improve physical function, physical activity, nutritional status and reduction of depressive symptoms. It verified the effectiveness of this programme in helping to prevent frailty, maintain functional independence of older people and improve their quality of life.

This proposal for physiotherapeutic intervention based on MACP focuses on an active kinesitherapy scheme with frequency, intensity and complexity suitable for older adults who require long-term care, who live or not in residential care homes and who may or may not have dementia. This kinesitherapy scheme focuses on a training routine that is easy to apply and can be managed by the caregiver.

3.1.2. Long-term care

Normally people think of ageing at home, living their golden years peacefully, but some ageing processes, with deterioration in physical or psychological health, lead to the elderly requiring family or professional care at home or in a nursing home. Long-term care are procedures or processes that are applied at home or in a specialised centre for the care needs of the elderly. They are based on two principles: firstly, when there is physical but not intellectual deterioration, despite the limitations, the older adult maintains a life project and has the right to a life of well-being, plenitude and respect. Secondly, it occurs when the older adult presents a psychological and cognitive deterioration that can be static or progressive. The older adult requires adequate care and it is necessary to adopt measures that optimise the physical and mental capacities that remain intact and compensate for the deficits due to their cognitive deterioration through the attention and support of their environment, generating a sense of well-being (WHO, 2015).

At present, there are homes and staff trained to provide care according to the comorbidities, pathologies or needs required by the elderly. They are based on the fundamental objective of taking care of health and that the person has a dignified and quality old age. Therefore, long-term caregivers should consider guidelines for the care of a person such as; the type of disease that afflicts the older adult, whether this disease is degenerative or not, the mental state if there is presence of stress, dementia, psychological or social alterations, the degree of independence of the older adult in their daily activities

The place where the older adult lives must meet standards to prevent falls, mobility problems and meet basic needs. There are four levels of action to ensure that people's basic needs are met: accessibility, safety, homeliness and personalisation. Accessibility, it must be a suitable place, in which mobility, communication, visualisation and accessibility to all spaces do not present difficulties and are not dangerous for the user. Safety, in the residence, modifications must be made to the furniture and distribution so that the spaces are safe places and avoid places that could cause falls or injuries. Homely feeling, it helps the person to have a relationship of belonging with the environment, controlling or avoiding periods of anxiety or depression in the older adult. Personalisation, it should be a private space with relevance to the characteristics of the person, the user's room should include memories of family, hobbies, friends and tastes (Moreno, 2017).

In the study by Goudriaan et al, (2021) revealed favourable results on adequate indoor lighting, referring to the reduction of depressive symptoms and the facilitation of spatial orientation. With regard to challenging behaviour, we only found indications for a very specific light intervention to decrease agitation.

3.1.3. Reminiscences

The influence of social, family and individual situations across the lifespan can lead to structural changes in the ageing process of older adults, while influencing health and well-being (Bech et al., 2019). Reminiscence benefits cognitive health, boosting memory, remembering influences the ability to think, learn and remember clearly.

Reminiscence is a non-pharmacological therapy used especially for people with dementia, who have difficulty remembering recent events, but find it easy to recall their past, especially their childhood and youth. The person can connect with the memory of skills and abilities acquired at a younger age, information that the health professional will welcome to develop and encourage.

Older adults use recalling events, feelings and thoughts from the past, in order to create and facilitate feelings of pleasure, and to improve quality of life or to adapt to situations. Reminiscence can play a positive role in improving quality of life, memory performance, awareness and health status when applied as a psychological treatment. Older people returning to the past through their memories can help people achieve greater balance in their lives (Kousha et al., 2021).

Reminiscence should be guided by a professional, who will help the older adult to interpret, explore and examine their emotions, memories, generating positive thoughts and overcoming episodes of the past. Being guided by a professional will help to avoid anxiety and depression.

In MACP, reminiscence is important, as it generates important memories in the person, this information is captured in the user's life history, a document that integrates memories, way of life, hobbies, experiences, expectations, achievements, failures written as a story, describing a unique and unrepeatable being.

Music as part of the reminiscence process is important for remembering, the study by Lopez et al. (2020) on autobiographical emotional induction in older people through popular songs identified that music produces different effects according to age. Enculturation may be an important mediating factor in emotionality and memory. The study design yielded a relatively high level of memory specificity and emotional positivity.

3.1.4. Life History

Life history is a method used in gerontology as a complementary element for intervention and care of the older adult, it is a bibliography narrated by the older adult about events in his or her life, in people with dementia this story is told or corroborated by family and friends. In the study by El Haj and Gallouj (2019) on self-defined memories in normal ageing, they conclude that the updating of one's identity across the lifespan, at least in normal ageing, may be related to the formation and retrieval of self-defined memories, memories that lead to the creation of narrative scripts, which in themselves serve as ingredients for "chapters" across the lifespan.

In another study by Bluck and McAdams (2021) on the vulnerability of older adults to the pandemic, they found older adults to be emotionally stable at the societal level, and consider that, in conducting life histories, the picture that emerges is one of older adults with the potential to show considerable psychosocial strength despite the adversities of the pandemic (Lind et al, 2021).

Active ageing

In a changing world, access to innovations and improvements in health, technology and food, with programmes to maintain optimal health status, has changed people's lives, improving conditions and increasing life expectancy, leading to an ageing phenomenon. Increasing life expectancy and a larger ageing population create economic, social and health challenges that must be addressed by health care providers, family members and society (WHO, 2012).

The WHO (2002) modified the concept of Healthy Ageing as a process of promoting and maintaining functional capacity that enables well-being in old age. It suggests that ageing is not the absence of disease, it is maintaining a healthy life with programmed medical monitoring, avoiding complications of comorbidities, predisposition to diseases due to hereditary or genetic factors, or alterations due to acquired diseases.

The WHO guidelines (Bull et al, 2020), reaffirms the recommendations published by WHO (2010), in which it reports that physical activity is better than nothing for optimal health outcomes and a reduction in sedentary behaviours. It stresses the importance of regular aerobic and muscle-strengthening activities.

Five guidelines are necessary to achieve active ageing (Government of Spain, 2011).

- Good health, the programme is based on promoting healthy eating, scheduled medical check-ups, monitoring of vital signs, regular clinical examinations, control of daily medication intake.
- Good physical functioning, physical exercise at least three times a week, maintaining physical activity in the daily routine. A physical activity programme can be carried out under the guidance and supervision of professionals.
- Good mental functioning, intellectual and cognitive activities to maintain and improve mental and learning capacity.
- To be independent and autonomous: in the daily routine to carry out activities in an autonomous and independent manner, in order to prevent functional limitation and dependence.
- Social links and participation, to avoid problems of depression or abandonment, it is important to have contact with family and friends and to carry out group activities.

Daily exercise in older adults is essential for active ageing, as demonstrated by the 3-month walking programme in older adults by Hsu et al. (2021), which showed significant improvements in body composition (BMI), lower limb strength and performance, balance and mobility function.

3.2.1Body outline

Modifications in the older adult's body schema can cause difficulties in independence and in performing activities of daily living.

Body schema is the basis of knowledge, idea or personal conception that the individual has of his or her body. The conception of the body schema is fundamental for the older adult to have a perception of his or her body. In order to improve or recover the body schema, it is necessary to work on laterality, attitude, relaxation and breathing.

Laterality, it is aimed at working on the schemes of up-down, left-right, the work of improving the work of the dominant and non-dominant side. Attitude, is the non-voluntary modification that the body undergoes due to internal and external causes, which affects muscle tone. Muscle tone can be seen on three levels, resting tone, attitude tone and action tone. In the *resting tone* the body is relaxed, at rest, without the presence of degrees of tension. In the *attitude tone,* in this state the muscle tone prepares us for movement, ready to react to a stimulus. In the *action tone,* the muscle tone increases in order to make an effort. Relaxation, different relaxation methods are used to improve the body scheme. Breathing, the proper control of breathing helps the knowledge of the body, it goes together with the relaxation technique.

When assessing posture, movement and strength in the older adult, the therapist shall record in the clinical history whether there are alterations in the resident's muscle tone that cause alterations in the resident's body schema.

3.2.2 Coordination

The resident with adequate coordination increases efficiency in the reception of information on body position, through the work of the central nervous system, with adequate communication with the muscular system, to maintain systematic control of movement. Coordination should be worked on in a schematic, continuous and complex way, and the exercises should be practical, accessible, adaptable and variable so that the older adult can perform the task in an optimal way.

When working on coordination, consideration should be given to:

- To develop or improve the manual-ocular scheme.
- To control the handling of space-time, to improve the perception of distance and the constant relationship between movement and

rhythm, to acquire notions of before, during and after, of simultaneity and succession, of perception of pauses, rhythms and durations.

- Perceptual constancy is a set of learning processes based on the constant stimulation of complex movements in different activities. It can be improved and mechanised with rhythmic gymnastics.

Comprehensive geriatric assessment

In the guidelines of active ageing, prevention and medical monitoring is important for good health, therefore the interdisciplinary team should perform a comprehensive geriatric assessment (GGA), which is an instrument that allows, together with the clinical assessment of the older adult patient, to integrate knowledge of the clinical, psychological, mental and social spheres, which enables a broad and clear view of the patient's situation, the main objective is to improve the accuracy of the diagnosis, as well as to identify related problems not previously diagnosed.

Conducting an IGV gives us clear and precise goals (D'Hyver, 2017):

- Generate new diagnoses, by making a global assessment of the human body without focusing only on the signs and symptoms of the current disease, it is possible to find medical problems that were not considered and that affect the state of health.

- With a comprehensive diagnosis, appropriate treatment can be carried out, thus reducing the number of days spent in health care institutions.
- With a VGI, the user is treated by an interdisciplinary medical team, lowering health care costs and reducing drug treatment.
- Upon discharge from the hospital and after a functional, cognitive and affective evaluation, optimal diagnoses and treatment are obtained, which focuses on the user's overall state of health.
- With the application of a VGI and the assessment of an interdisciplinary team, the user will have a better quality.

IGV should be managed by the interdisciplinary team and will include anamnesis and physical examination (D'Hyver, 2017):

- Head: assessment of temporal arteries, mouth (dental status, prostheses, mycosis, tumours), eyes (visual capacity and presence of cataracts, entropion and ectropion), hearing capacity.
- Neck: presence of goitre, lymphadenopathy, jugular ingurgitation, murmurs, cervical stiffness.
- Chest: cardiac and pulmonary auscultation, breast palpation in women and presence of spinal deformities (dorsal kyphosis).
- Abdomen: same as adult (inspection, palpation, percussion and auscultation).

- Rectal examination: for haemorrhoids, faecal impaction and prostate examination in men.
- Limbs: muscle strength and tone, presence of pulses and reflexes, and intentional search for oedema or joint deformities (including toes).
- Neurological: Speech disorders, tremor, rigidity, akinesia, balance, gait, sensation.
- Skin: trophic lesions, ulcers, tumours.

In addition, a Functional Assessment, Katz index (1963, cited in D'Hyver, 2017), Lawton and Brody index (1993, as cited in D'Hyver, 2017); SPPB Physical Performance; Gait and Balance; Nutritional Assessment; and Affective Assessment will be included. This comprehensive assessment provides a global view of the person, their physical, mental, psychological and social state of health, in order for the interdisciplinary team to provide comprehensive treatment.

In the study of Medication costs in older patients: before and after comprehensive geriatric assessment by Unutmaz et al. (2018) showed that IGV could reduce the prevalence of polypharmacy in older adults. In addition, this will have beneficial effects on economic parameters due to decreased medication-related healthcare costs.

3.4. Physiotherapy

According to the guidelines for active ageing, physiotherapy is a means of support to achieve this. Physiotherapy plays an important role in the recovery of the individual to improve or maintain their independence and perform activities of daily living. Physiotherapy is the art and science of physical treatment; that is, the set of methods, actions and techniques, which through the application of physical means cure, prevent diseases, promote health, recover, enable and readapt people affected by somatic dysfunctions or those who wish to maintain an adequate level of health (COLFISIOCV, 2021).

According to the VGI, physiotherapy is applied in a preventive, curative or palliative way, intervening with the application of techniques and methods so that the person can carry out the activities of daily living with independence and autonomy.

3.4.1. Physiotherapeutic Assessment

The physiotherapeutic evaluation is carried out through a process of dialogue, interacting with the patient, with the objective application of tests, scales and clinical tests to make an adequate diagnosis , set goals and treatment times for optimal rehabilitation (Mantilla, 2018).

The therapist will carry out an assessment according to his/her level of observation, expertise and experience, and will perform a detailed assessment of the individual, determining his/her deficits, residual capacities, neuromusculoskeletal alterations, degree of difficulty in performing different movements and loss of agility in activities of daily living. With the diagnosis developed by the interdisciplinary team, the therapist will determine the type of assessment, tests and instruments to be used to give an interpretation and make a therapeutic diagnosis, prognosis and clinical decision-making for the implementation of rehabilitation programmes (Mantilla, 2018). By analysing the clinical history and assessment carried out by the therapist, short- and long-term goals will be drawn up, the number of sessions and the type of treatment will be determined.

The evaluation will be recorded in the physiotherapeutic clinical history, consisting of: anamnesis, clinical diagnosis, medication, physical examination, musculoskeletal system, neuromuscular functional system, with the analysis of this information the objectives, treatment plan, observations and recommendations will be determined.

The anamnesis is the section of the clinical history where personal, social and vocational information is detailed, evaluating the environment and a vision of the patient's psychological structure. will detail the clinical data, the illnesses suffered, the medication habitually used, the history and onset of the symptoms or signs of the current illness, examinations carried out. In other words, a medical history preceding the current illness will be detailed (Kottke and Lehmann, 2002).

Clinical diagnosis is a process that concludes after evaluation of the clinical picture, its function is to define the disease affecting a patient. The clinical picture is made up of three interrelated elements: the syndrome, the disease and the context. The syndrome is the group of signs and symptoms presented by the patient from the onset of the disease, the disease is determined by the relationship of signs and symptoms presented by the patient, and the context is the relationship of the social, economic and psychological environment in which the person suffering from the disease develops (Capurro and Rada, 2007). The physiotherapist starts from the clinical diagnosis to determine the type of therapeutic assessment to be carried out on the patient, and at the same time will provide a guideline for a global approach to the problems or deficits that the patient may present.

In terms of medication, reference is made to the drugs that are administered to the patient to maintain the balance and work of the body. The therapist collects information on the basis of these parameters to determine treatment schedules.

Physical examination, the musculoskeletal physical examination will assess pain, deformity, weakness, limitation of movement and stiffness. The physical examination has three functions (Kottke and Lehamann, 2002)

1. See alignment of a structure, if there are deviations, deformations, movement and its biomechanics is normal.

2. Find problems secondary to the disease that may indirectly affect the structure.
3. Assess the residual capacity of systems or parts of systems not affected by the disease.

In the physical examination, the therapist will evaluate the skin, if there are bony prominences, vasomotor alterations, lesions, scars or dermatitis. Sensitivity will be evaluated if the patient presents alterations, if there are anaesthetised areas, superficial pain, deep pain. For the musculoskeletal system, the functional unit is the joint and its associated structures: the synovial membrane and capsule, ligaments and surrounding muscles (Kottke and Lehmann, 2002). When assessing the musculoskeletal system we will determine abnormalities in shape, alignment that may cause conditions affecting the patient, the assessment will include inspection, palpation, passive range of motion, stability, active range of motion, muscle strength.

On inspection, the joint is examined for symmetry in contour and size. On palpation, the source of pain, contractures, swellings, bony masses or synovial effusions are located. In passive range of motion, the patient is relaxed, and the therapist performs the joint movement and determines whether there are any limitations in movement. In stability, different tests are used to assess whether the cause of the pathological problem is caused by the muscle, capsule or ligament. Active range of motion, the therapist asks the patient to perform a specific movement and verifies if there is pain or limitation of movement. Muscle strength is determined according to the Daniels test, which will indicate the degree of muscle strength of the patient.

The Neuromuscular Functional Test defines the patient's ability to perform daily activities. It determines the patient's functional status. Tests are carried out in which the patient will demonstrate their dexterity or deficit. It assesses sitting and standing balance, transfers, feeding ability, dressing ability, personal hygiene ability, walking (Kottke and Lehmann, 2002).

Balance in the sitting position, if the patient masters or maintains this position, he/she will be able to perform transfer activities. Transfers are assessed from the change of position from decubitus, prone to supinc and latcral, sitting, standing and walking. Balancc in thc standing position is a requirement for walking, balance is assessed with and without support, support on one leg and balance reaction; difficulty or inability to perform these tests will suggest problems at the vestibular level that will be assessed by the specialist. Feeding ability, hand-mouth coordination is assessed. Dressing ability, the patient's coordination when dressing is assessed. Capacity for personal hygiene, the patient's independence is assessed when carrying out personal hygiene activities, and the level of difficulty he/she has when carrying them out. Ambulation, assessing the patient's balance when standing and whether there are any difficulties in the phases of walking (Bernal et al, 2006).

In order to carry out the physiotherapeutic evaluation for the present intervention proposal, the following factors were analysed: age group, type of activity of daily living, social, psychological and physical conditions. Therefore, when evaluating the factors, the following tests and evaluations were determined: Postural Test, Daniels Test, Tinetti Scale, Berg Scale, Balance Test, Walking Speed Test, Chair Rising Test, Rosow- Breslau Scale.

As for the physiotherapeutic plan, this section of the clinical history will analyse the data found in the assessment and determine the short and long term objectives. The recommendations given by the interdisciplinary team and the patient's comorbidities will be considered. With the objectives drawn up, the number of sessions and the treatment to be followed will be established, according to the pathology and evaluation, physical means, electrotherapy, kinesitherapy, instrumental manipulation will be applied. In this intervention proposal, three types of activities are applied: active assisted kinesitherapy, coordination and balance exercises and circuits.

Kinesiotherapy shall consist of warm-up, stretching, strengthening, balance and coordination exercises. The physiotherapeutic evaluation will determine the duration, frequency, rate of progression and intensity of each exercise. The duration is determined by the patient's physical condition and can last between 10 to 30 minutes. Frequency is determined by the patient's daily routine, level of physical activity and comorbidities. In the group of exercises proposed, we started with a 5-minute routine and increased daily until reaching 30 minutes of activity. The pace of progression will be in accordance with the patient's comorbidities, mental and physical state. Intensity, will be progressively with assisted active kinesitherapy, as the exercise is mastered by the older adult, will pass to free active kinesitherapy and we will finish with resisted active kinesitherapy. When 50% of the treatment has been completed, the patient's condition should be assessed and it should be verified whether the objectives set are being met.

In observations and recommendations, the guidelines and guidelines given to the patient to perform exercises, the number of repetitions and suggestions for performing activities of daily living without difficulty are written down.

3.4.2. Kinesiotherapy

It is an important axis for physiotherapy, it is a set of techniques and procedures based on movement that is applied in physiotherapy for the treatment and prevention of diseases that produce problems or alterations in the locomotor system and the muscular system. It helps us to improve or maintain trophism and muscle power (Fernández and Melián, 2013).

The objectives of kinesitherapy are linked to the objectives set by the therapist, thus helping us to improve the body's structure, avoid and reduce the retraction of muscles, tendons or ligaments. On the other hand, it prevents joint stiffness, helps us to improve or recover normal joint movement. With the application of exercises, vicious attitudes and postures are corrected. By improving muscle toning and correcting vicious attitudes, relaxation and pain reduction are achieved (De las Peñas and Ortiz 2013).

By applying kinesitherapy as a maintenance and preventive technique, muscle function is improved and muscle atrophy, fibrosis, venous and lymphatic stasis, which can be caused by periods of immobilisation, is avoided. Kinesitherapy improves the performance of the older adult in activities of daily living.

Kinesitherapy, when applied in a targeted and appropriate manner, has a beneficial effect on the human body. It optimises cardiovascular and respiratory work. It has a positive effect on the psychological, emotional and physiological level. The stimulation of exercise increases the bone remodelling process. At the same time the application of active resisted kinesitherapy hypertrophies muscle fibres

The basic principles of kinesitherapy provide essential guidelines for exercise.

- The resident should be in a comfortable position. The therapist should be in an ergonomic posture to avoid fatigue and spinal problems.

- Patient-therapist trust, the patient must understand the guidelines of the exercise and at the same time trust the therapist to indicate if they feel they are not being treated with respect.
- The therapist must consider that each patient is unique, and therefore the exercise must be individually mapped out.
- Respect for pain: pain generates defensive phenomena in the patient, such as increased muscle tension or compensations that may go against the desired objective.
- Treatment progression: frequency of sessions, duration of treatments and dosage within each of the mobilisations, according to the pathology and improvement of each patient.

Kinesitherapy is classified as passive and active. In passive kinesitherapy, the therapist moves the joint without the patient having to exert any effort. In active kinesitherapy, the patient performs the movement under the guidance of the therapist. Active kinesitherapy can be either free active or assisted active. On the other hand, in free active kinesitherapy, the patient has the muscle strength, balance and coordination to perform the exercise without problems. Finally, in active assisted kinesitherapy, the patient does not have adequate muscle strength, balance and coordination and requires support from the therapist to perform the exercise.

Active kinesiotherapy encompasses various methods, techniques and processes that are applied to the user with a prior physiotherapeutic assessment. One of the methods applied is that of Frenklen (1946, as cited in Kottke and Lehmann, 2002) and a series of coordination training circuits. Frenklen's method consists of systematic and graded exercises that are used for the treatment of incoordination. The application of this method assists the voluntary regulation of movement by using whatever part of the sensory mechanism has remained intact, usually the senses of sight, hearing and touch, to compensate for the loss of kinaesthetic sensation. Its principles are: concentration, precision and repetition. Concentration, when performing the exercise, the person must not have any distracting elements, their senses must be focused on the action of the movement. Precision: when performing the movement, there should be no mistakes, therefore the person has no time limit to perform the exercise. The repetitions, the more repetitions without failures, the more the brain will record the exercise, thus mastering the movement (Romero, 2016).

Its objective is to regulate the movement, the person, by performing controlled and exact repetitions of an exercise, masters it, which generates confidence and security. The application of this method is progressive and the complexity of the movements increases. It starts with minimal repetitions and is applied progressively. The progression of the exercise must comply with several parameters: the speed, amplitude and complexity of the exercise must be alternated. As the user masters the exercise it should be modified in difficulty and not in power. Simple exercises with large joint amplitude should be started and replaced with finer movements that require greater precision. Initially, the exercise should be performed with eyes open, then with eyes closed. The exercise should not be strenuous, should not cause fatigue or generate a high muscular effort.

With the initial assessment, the physiotherapist will determine the degree of disability or difficulty the user has, and will draw up a schedule of re-education exercises. The sequence can be supine to lateral, prone, sitting, standing and walking. As the user practices the exercises, it will become easier to master them. Avoid intense exercises that cause fatigue, dizziness or tiredness.

Regarding the coordination training circuits, they are a group of interconnected, sequential exercises, with rest periods, established by the therapist with a duration of 10 to 20 minutes that will group warm-up, stretching, coordination, balance and walking exercises. The therapist should provide reassurance, confidence and explain each point of the circuit in a simple manner. If necessary, the therapist will perform the circuit first so that the older adult understands the activity to be performed. The therapist can guide or support the older adult with his or her hand to reassure him or her in the execution of the exercise.

The work in the circuit is individualised, the duration and modifications will be made according to the patient's comorbidities. The user will improve their concentration, agility, balance, mental state and we will help them to carry out their daily activities more easily.

When choosing a circuit, the level of complexity of the activity with specific guidelines and times, the method to be used, the objectives to be achieved, the resources required, the experiences to be developed while doing the activity and the evaluation at the end of the circuit should be considered.

In order to design the circuits, we must outline the objectives with a specific purpose, focusing on the development of the older adult's capacity. The construction of tasks according to their own structure and capacities can be divided into sub-tasks, which must be related to each other in order to work on the progression, complexity, increase of elements and duration of the circuit.

In order to achieve a goal, it is important to know the elements that influence the performance of tasks, the factors that affect the older adult can be biological, psychological and social. The therapist assesses the factors before performing the activity or task and may modify it before each intervention. Modification of tasks should be compatible with the goals set.

Each session should be structured in three parts, the first or preparatory, the second or basic, and the third of relaxation. The first or preparatory part is based on the warm-up and stretching phase, which prepares the body to activate the body and prepare it for the effort activity, the approximate time for this activity is 5 to 10 minutes. It is considered to be divided into two parts, the first is passive with breathing exercises to oxygenate and relax the body, the second part is active, a short walk and stretching exercises will be carried out progressively without the patient making a great effort.

The second or basic part, in this phase the person will make their maximum effort, the average time to be used is 15 to 30 minutes, the time, speed, strength and resistance of the activity must be considered, it will depend on the physical and psychological characteristics and the illnesses that each older adult presents in the application of the activity.

The third or final phase, this phase is the clama or adaptation of the exercise to relax and reduce the intensity of the activity, this session usually lasts between 5 to 10 minutes. Relaxation techniques, breathing exercises and stretching are applied.

It is important to observe the behaviour of the person while performing the exercise, suspending or taking rest periods if dizziness, tachycardia, fatigue, dyspnoea or tiredness are present. When working with older adults on coordination circuits, the therapist should consider that modifications should be made while performing the series of exercises to avoid frustration or periods of anxiety in the patient. The complexity of the exercise should go from low to high, the therapist cannot leave the patient to perform the exercise alone and should be at the side guiding and alert to a loss of balance that may cause a fall (Garcia, 2013).

In physiotherapy, appropriate kinesiotherapy for the elderly is based on the aerobic capacity and medical history of this age group. A kinesiotherapy programme for older people should consider short periods of exercise alternating with regular rest breaks, it is important to perform exercises that involve as many muscle groups as possible with minimal effort. In order to facilitate learning, recall and execution, complicated activities should be avoided (Kottke and Lehmann, 2002).

The main advantages of physical activity at older ages (Government of Spain, 2011) are:

- Stimulated physical activity improves and preserves muscle trophism and bone mineral density, preventing muscle atrophy due to disuse and osteoporosis.
- Increases aerobic capacity for exertion and improves quality of life.
- It reduces the risk of cardiovascular disease. It also reduces the risk of cardiovascular problems caused by smoking or hypercholesterolemia.

- It improves water balance and thus prevents diseases such as diabetes mellitus and obesity.
- Helps relaxation and elimination of toxins, thus reducing anxiety and depression problems. Improving mental activity.
- It collaborates in physiotherapy processes, playing a positive role in joint, respiratory, traumatological, vascular and post-surgical rehabilitation.

In the study of physical exercise for the prevention and treatment of Alzheimer's disease by De la rosa et al, (2020), they conclude that promoting lifestyle changes in the pre-symptomatic and pre-dementia stages of the disease may have the potential to delay one third of dementias worldwide

On the other hand, the study by Hortobágyi et al. (2021) indicates that increased motor performance is often accompanied by neuroplastic adaptations in the central nervous system for improved function in the older adult. He recommends a systematic analysis with new approaches to corroborate the functional relevance of endurance training-induced neuroplasticity.

3.4.3 Physiotherapy from the ACP

As health professionals we are trained to meet the basic needs of the person, which are encompassed in the 5 basic needs: comfort, identity, attachment, occupation and inclusion. Comfort is related to establishing a relationship of warmth, respect and concern for the older adult. Identity, knowing their history, their preferences, dislikes, feelings and thoughts. Attachment, when carrying out the treatment we develop bonds or commitments with the user. Occupation, when carrying out the treatment and while the kinesiotherapy is being carried out, we should try to make the user feel useful and active. Inclusion, if it is feasible to carry out group activities once a week so that users feel part of a community (Moreno, 2017).

The MACP-based approach to physiotherapy should have several guidelines:

- The physiotherapy sessions must be individual and guided by the therapist, the person is considered as a unique and unrepeatable being, therefore the attention is based on satisfying the particular needs of the user.
- Older adults with a history of dementia should be treated with respect. It is important to inquire about their life history with the family and the interdisciplinary care team in order to have a comprehensive approach to their health problems.
- As each person is unique and unrepeatable, it is necessary with the physiotherapeutic assessment to make a therapy schedule appropriate to the needs, requirements and limitations of each user.

- Once the physiotherapy schedule is established, it should be socialised with the older adult for feedback or modifications to the exercise programme.
- When carrying out the therapeutic intervention it is important to consider the recommendations of the interdisciplinary team.
- Once or twice a week, music to the user's liking is included in the therapy.
- Give recommendations and guidelines for performing the routines to the caregiver or auxiliary of the geriatric centre.

The 9-week programme of aerobic and strength training improves cognitive and motor function in dementia patients by Bossers (2015) showed that compared to a control group with no exercise, a combination of aerobic and strength training is more effective than aerobic training alone in slowing cognitive and motor decline in dementia patients. No mediating effects were found between improvements in cognitive function through improved motor function.

The dementia and physical activity trial of moderate- to high-intensity exercise training for people with dementia by Lamb et al. (2018) showed that a moderate- to high-intensity aerobic and strength exercise training programme does not slow cognitive decline in people with mild to moderate dementia. The exercise training programme improved physical fitness, but there were no notable improvements in other clinical outcomes.

Moreover, in the study by Morris et al. (2017) based on aerobic exercise for Alzheimer's disease: a pilot randomised controlled trial conducted in early Alzheimer's disease showed that aerobic exercise is associated with benefits in functional capacity. Exercise-related gains in cardiorespiratory fitness were associated with improved memory performance and reduced hippocampal atrophy, suggesting that gains in cardiorespiratory fitness may be important in generating brain benefits.

Another intervention is Asmidawati et al.'s (2014) home-based exercise to improve turning performance and mobility among community-dwelling older adults: protocol for a randomised controlled trial, showed the results of this study will provide useful information for clinicians on the types of exercises to improve turning ability in older people at increased risk of falls and the effectiveness of these exercises to improve outcomes. Given the importance of balance for the independence and safety of older people, and the negative effect of age and health problems on balance ability, exercise has been a widely researched intervention to improve balance and reduce the risk of falls. A Cochrane review reported that multicomponent group exercise, which generally includes resistance and balance training, reduced the rate of falls by 22% and the risk of falls by 17% in adults aged 60 years and older.

4. Objectives

4.1. General Objective

To design a proposal for physiotherapeutic intervention in elderly people in geriatric centres based on the MACP.

4.2. Specific Objectives

- Draw up a care and co-morbidities scheme based on the person's medical history.
- Know the person's life history and preferences.
- To get to know relevant aspects of the resident through their relatives.
- Analyse life histories with the interdisciplinary team
- Designing personalised physiotherapy sessions
- Implement the personalised sessions at the centre
- Assessing the results of the experience

5. Methodology

5.1 . Type of study

The present work is an intervention proposal for elderly people living in geriatric centres based on the principles of MACP

It is based on the analysis of the literature related to PCA and physiotherapy for the development of the programme. And its application in a residential centre for the elderly is proposed. The collaboration of the centre's interdisciplinary team is required to collect data that will help to adapt a physiotherapy clinical history and to create a kinesitherapy schedule for each person. And, through the use of semi-structured interviews, relevant autobiographical data will be collected from the residents to create a life history.

5.2 Participants

The intervention is aimed at elderly people living in geriatric centres. It is mainly aimed at working with residents with dementia and balance and coordination problems. Although it is open to residents without significant cognitive impairment who require attention in the Physiotherapy Service. Excluded from the intervention are people who do not wish to participate and residents whose carers do not wish them to participate, and who do not sign the informed consent form.

The design is applied to a sample of 6 residents of a geriatric centre in Ecuador, in the province of Pichincha, Sangolquí canton.

5.3 Characteristics of the centre

Oasis de Plata is a Residential Club for the elderly is the centre where the practices of the Master's Degree in Gerontology and Person-Centred Care of the International University of Valencia have been carried out. Its mission is to share and be reborn together with the elderly and their wisdom, to harmonise our lives through recreation and the reactivation of emotions and sensations. Its vision is to be a centre of attention and care for the elderly in order to achieve harmony in life, through a space for integration, recreation and interaction.

As for its facilities, the centre is a 2-storey house with individual en-suite rooms for the 6 older adults, it has a living room, 1 social bathroom, a dining room, a kitchen, a rest area where they can sunbathe in the mornings, and green space where they can walk, as well as fruit trees, canaries and rabbits. The centre offers day care, permanent care and temporary care.

5.4. Materials-Instruments

5.4.1 Medical history

The resident's medical history provided information on health and psychological status, the recommendations of the interdisciplinary team, pharmacological indications and physiotherapeutic assessment. This information indicated the strengths and limitations of the resident to make an individual scheme of physiotherapeutic intervention based on the Person-Centred Care model.

In the physiotherapeutic evaluation proposed for this study, the following tests and assessments are determined:

- Postural Test (Mantilla, 2018) allows us to measure our body posture. It helps us to detect any deformity in the body. It evaluates the anterior, posterior and lateral view.
- Daniels Test (1946, as cited in Kottke and Lehmann, 2002) allows measuring muscle strength, by muscle groups and individually, determining a scale in grades ranging from 0 to 5, where grade 0 is absence of muscle contraction and no joint movement and grade 5 is muscle contraction overcoming resistance and full joint range.
- Tinetti Scale (1986, as cited in Mantilla, 2018), assesses a person's walking ability and balance and determines their risk of falling.
- Berg Scale (1992, as cited in Mantilla, 2018), used to measure the patient's ability to sit, stand, extend the arms without losing balance, stand on one leg and turn.
- Balance test (Mantilla, 2018), consists of assessing and timing the patient's ability to stand in different positions: with feet side by side, in semi-tandem and tandem position; if the patient is able to maintain the position for at least 10 seconds, he/she does not have balance problems.
- Walking speed test (Kottke and Lehmann, 2002), at a distance of 4 metres the patient is asked to walk and the time taken to complete the distance is timed.

- Test of getting up from the chair (Mantilla, 2018), the seated patient is asked to stand up with his arms folded over his chest. If the patient is able to perform it, he/she must perform 5 repetitions of the exercise and the time it takes to perform it is taken.
- Rosow-Breslau Scale (1966, as cited in Mantilla, 2018), consists of several items, but we rely on the mobility item, in which we assess walking, activities at home and going up and down stairs.

Once the different assessments have been applied to each user, the short and long term objectives are determined in order to draw up the treatment plan.

The treatment plan was applied individually, with an approximate time of 20 to 30 minutes per user. Evaluations were carried out every 3 days to determine the evolution of the application of kinesitherapy in the older adults.

5.4.2. Semi-structured interview with the resident

Interviews were conducted randomly and individually with each resident. The scheme of questions:

- As he likes to be called.
- The length of stay in the centre.
- The activities he carried out during his rest hours, before entering the Centre.

- Work activity, office hours or activities at home.
- Hobbies and whether he/she was interested in any sport.
- Illnesses suffered, surgeries performed.
- If you are visually or hearing impaired. If you use assistive devices (glasses or hearing aids).
- If you are aware of your current health status.
- Difficulties in performing ADLs at the Centre.
- The activities you like to participate in.
- Activities that are not to their liking.
- Presence of difficulties in walking or occupational therapy activities.
- The music you like, for listening or activities.
- The activities that you would like to see increased at the Centre or that you would like to do.
- Prefer to do the activity alone or in a group.

5.4.3. Interview of the interdisciplinary team

By conducting a dialogue with the interdisciplinary team, a global vision of the resident was achieved, and according to each speciality, an approach and recommendations were obtained for a positive result in the intervention. The outline of questions to each of the members of the interdisciplinary team was based on:

- In the field or speciality in which it operates.
- Time spent working at the Gerontological Centre.
- Diagnosis and medication applied to each of the users.
- Recommendations on care and work for each older adult.
- How often do you carry out a check-up or intervention with older adults?
- The achievements of their intervention and experiences with residents.
- A weekly dialogue with the interdisciplinary team takes place to learn about the residents' health and psychological condition.

5.4.4. Life history

It is important to recognise the resident as a unique, independent person with a past with experiences, joys, memories, hobbies and sorrows, and for this reason it was recommended that the geriatric centre create a document with the resident's life history. In the interview with the resident, a dialogue about memories and experiences was developed.

For the implementation of the life history in the residents, several interviews were carried out during the internship period, these conversations were conducted while walking in the garden or when people were sunbathing in the morning, it is emphasised that the interviews were individual, with discretion, strict confidentiality, respecting the space and with due care for the complexity of the answers.

The questions generated from users and carers were:

- Family information: place of birth, parents, siblings, aunts, uncles, cousins, etc.
- Childhood information: where you grew up, memories as a child, whether you played pranks, names of your friends, relationship of your parents.
- Academic information: where you studied, school, college, university, experiences, academic memories, best friends.
- Information: hobbies, travels, memories, friends, joys and sorrows, experiences of your youth and maturity.
- Partner information; if married, who you married, how you met, children, grandchildren, names, experiences, experiences, memories.
- Music and sports: whether you like it or not, what sport you used to play, what music you like, whether you dance or not. Music that brings back memories.
- What projects do you have in your life, how do you feel at the moment?

5.4 Data collection procedure

In order to take a physiotherapeutic clinical history, the recommendations of the gerontological centre staff and relevant data from the life history of each user were included. Based on this assessment, a physiotherapeutic objective was drawn up for each patient, and a programme of coordination and balance exercises was then carried out accordingly.

Before collecting the data, a consent form was requested from the Gerontology Centre (Appendix 1.) and another for the family members or representatives of the users (Appendix 2.) so that they could approve the user's participation in this intervention proposal. Physiotherapeutic Clinical History (Annex 3.). Interviews were conducted with the interdisciplinary team of the gerontological centre, and interviews were conducted with the residents. Once the information in the physiotherapy clinical history had been coded, the treatment objectives were set for each resident.

The collection of information was divided into 6 sessions, the first session was a dialogue with the interdisciplinary team and the informed consent was sent to the relatives and the authorisation for data collection was sent to the Gerontology Centre, in the second session the first interview and anamnesis was carried out with each user and the clinical history was reviewed, the third session the postural test was carried out, the fourth session the Daniels test was carried out, Tinetti scale, the second interview was conducted with the users to discuss their personal and working life, the fifth session balance and coordination tests were conducted, the sixth session the third interview was conducted with the user about their life experiences and short or long term projects, the evaluation of the information collected in the user tests was conducted and the objectives and treatment were determined, from the seventh session balance and coordination exercises and circuits were conducted and a dialogue was held with the user about their tastes and preferences.

5.5 Intervention planning

The intervention is designed to take place over 2 months with daily sessions from Monday to Friday with each intervention lasting 30 minutes per resident.

During the first month and a half, informed consents are gathered, information is collected, and the sessions are designed. In the second fortnight of the second month, the sessions designed for each resident would be applied. However, due to confinements and restrictions derived from the pandemic, the intervention will only be applied for two weeks. Although this is a short period of time, feedback is expected to be collected in order to improve the present design.

The programme will be divided into: strengthening exercises twice a week, coordination exercises twice a week, once a week there will be a 20-minute walk with each resident to conduct a life history interview while listening to music to their liking. Each session will be planned according to the emotional, health and psychological state of the patient.

- OBJECTIVE: To improve muscular strength and coordination in walking.

The therapy is recommended for 2 months and will be divided into:

- Strengthening exercises twice a week.
- Coordination exercises 2 times a week.

Once a week, a 20-minute walk with each resident will take place to conduct a life history interview.

The duration of each intervention will be half an hour.

Each session will be planned according to the emotional, health and psychological state of the patient.

5.6.1. Distribution of exercises per day and week

WEEK 1

Day 1: Exercises will be performed in a seated position.

- Relaxation exercises, deep breathing with arm movements.
- Upper limb exercises (shoulder, elbow, wrist, fingers) 10 repetitions
- Lower limb exercises (hip, knee, ankle and toes) 10 repetitions

Day 2: Exercises will be performed in a seated position.

- Relaxation exercises, deep breathing with arm movements.
- The first circuit is carried out:

  Jigsaw: put togcthcr a 4-piccc jigsaw puzzlc
- Transfer: two buckets, one with balls and the other empty, place the balls from one bucket to the other.
- Stand up and sit down 4 times in a row

Day 3: Walk for 5 minutes at a time

Day 4: Exercises shall be performed in a seated position.

- Relaxation exercises, deep breathing with arm movements.
- Upper limb exercises (shoulder, elbow, wrist, fingers) 10 repetitions
- Lower limb exercises (hip, knee, ankle and toes) 10 repetitions

Day 5: Exercises will be performed in a sitting and standing position.

- Relaxation exercises, deep breathing with arm movements.
- The first circuit is carried out:
- Rings: rings placed on a pedestal, remove them with the right hand, place them on the table and replace them with the left hand.
- Transfer: two buckets one with balls and the other empty, each bucket must be on a different table, the resident must stand up and carry the ball from one bucket to the other.

- Walk in the stall for 5 minutes at a time.

WEEK 2

Day 1: Exercises will be performed in a standing position.

- Relaxation exercises, deep breathing with arm movements.
- Upper limb exercises (shoulder, elbow, wrist and fingers) 10 repetitions.
- Lower limb exercises (hip, knee, ankle and toes) 10 repetitions. Walking for 5 minutes at a time.

Day 2: Relaxation exercises, deep breathing with arm movements.

The circuit is made:

- Distance of 2 metres marked with a cone and 2 repetitions each, then proceed to the following exercises:
- Walk with support from the therapist and return back to the starting position.
- Get into lateral position and walk sideways back and forth.
- Stand on tiptoe 10 times
- Stand on your heels 10 times

Day 3: Walk for 10 minutes at a time, listening to music to the resident's liking.

Day 4: Exercises will be performed in a standing position.

- Relaxation exercises, deep breathing with arm movements.
- Upper limb exercises (shoulder, elbow, wrist and fingers) 10 repetitions.
- Lower limb exercises (hip, knee, ankle and toes) 10 repetitions. Walking for 5 minutes at a time.

Patient seated with a medium ball will perform 6 repetitions of the following exercises:

- Pass the ball from one hand to the other behind the back.
- Pass the ball from one hand to the other over the head.
- With the ball touching each of the toes.

<u>Day 5:</u> Relaxation exercises, deep breathing with arm movements.

- The following movements are performed to the resident's favourite song:
- Six steps forward, six steps back 5 repetitions
- Two side steps to the left, two side steps to the right, 10 repetitions.
- Walk in the stall, 30 seconds. This circuit will be repeated for the duration of the song.

WEEK 3

<u>Day 1:</u> Exercises will be performed in a standing position.

- Relaxation exercises, deep breathing with arm movements.

- Upper limb exercises (shoulder, elbow, wrist and fingers) 10 repetitions.
- Lower limb exercises (hip, knee, ankle and toes) 10 repetitions.
- Walk for 10 minutes at a time.
- Patient seated with a medium ball will perform 6 repetitions of the following exercises:
- Pass the ball from one hand to the other behind the back.
- Pass the ball from one hand to the other over the head.
- With the ball touching each of the toes.

Day 2: Relaxation exercises, deep breathing with arm movements.

The circuit is made:

- Distance of 3 metres marked with a cone0 and 2 repetitions each, then proceed to the following exercises:
- Walk with support from the therapist and return back to the starting position.
- Get into lateral position and walk sideways back and forth.
- Stand on tiptoe 10 times
- Stand on your heels 10 times
- Walk in a zigzag pattern twice.

Day 3: Take a walk for 20 minutes at a time, listening to music of the resident's liking and discussing the resident's memories.

<u>Day 4:</u> Exercises will be performed in a standing position.

- Relaxation exercises, deep breathing with arm movements.
- Upper limb exercises (shoulder, elbow, wrist and fingers) 10 repetitions.
- Lower limb exercises (hip, knee, ankle and toes) 10 repetitions. Walking for 10 minutes at a time, including a zigzag walk for a distance of 2 metres.
- Stand on tiptoe 10 times
- Stand on your heels 10 times
- Walk in a zigzag pattern twice.

<u>Day 5:</u> Relaxation exercises, deep breathing with arm movements.

Patient seated with a medium ball will perform 6 repetitions of the following exercises:

- Pass the ball from one hand to the other behind the back.
- Pass the ball from one hand to the other over the head.
- With the ball touching each of the toes.

The circuit to be performed will comprise 3 phases and 2 repetitions:

- Phase I: zigzag walk distance 2 metres
- Phase II: throw a ball and knock down pins that are 2 metres away.

- Phase III: 2 buckets, one with balls and one empty, transfer the balls from one bucket to the other.

WEEK 4

Day 1: Exercises will be performed in a standing position.

- Relaxation exercises, deep breathing with arm movements.
- Upper limb exercises (shoulder, elbow, wrist and fingers) 10 repetitions.
- Lower limb exercises (hip, knee, ankle and toes) 10 repetitions.

Patient seated with a medium ball will perform 6 repetitions of the following exercises:

- Pass the ball from one hand to the other behind the back.
- Pass the ball from one hand to the other over the head.
- With the ball touching each of the toes.
- Walk for 15 minutes at a time.

Day 2: Relaxation exercises, deep breathing with arm movements.

The circuit is made:

- Distance of 3 metres marked with a cone and 2 repetitions each, then proceed to the following exercises:
- Walk with support from the therapist and return back to the starting position.

- Get into lateral position and walk sideways back and forth.
- Stand on tiptoe 10 times
- Stand on your heels 10 times
- Walk in zigzag three times.

Day 3: Take a walk for 20 minutes at a time, listening to music to the resident's liking and discussing the resident's memories.

Day 4: Exercises will be performed in a standing position.

- Relaxation exercises, deep breathing with arm movements.
- Upper limb exercises (shoulder, elbow, wrist and fingers) 10 repetitions.
- Lower limb exercises (hip, knee, ankle and toes) 10 repetitions. Walking for 10 minutes at a time, including a zigzag walk for a distance of 2 metres.
- Stand on tiptoe 10 times
- Stand on your heels 10 times.

Day 5: Relaxation exercises, deep breathing with arm movements.

- Patient seated with a medium ball will perform 6 repetitions of the following exercises:
- Pass the ball from one hand to the other behind the back.
- Pass the ball from one hand to the other over the head.
- With the ball touching each of the toes.

The circuit to be performed will comprise 4 phases and 2 repetitions:

- Phase I: zigzag walk distance 2 metres, then a distance of one metre backwards, assisted by the therapist.
- Phase II: kicking a ball
- Phase III: 2 buckets, one with balls and one empty, with a separation distance of 2 metres, throw the balls from one bucket to the other.

6 Results

The present intervention proposal was divided into two parts, the first lasting 2 months with interviews once a week, the activities were the collection of information for the development of the Physiotherapeutic Clinical History based on the MACP, the Life History and the planning of the treatment for each resident, the second part was carried out for a period of two weeks from Monday to Friday with the application of the physiotherapeutic treatment to each resident. The time of application was shorter than planned due to changes resulting from the pandemic confinement situation. Nevertheless, it was possible to observe an improvement in the residents' muscle strength and coordination when performing activities. In turn, a better willingness to perform the exercises, with an appropriate state of mind.

There was one exception. A user who, due to his accelerated cognitive impairment due to Alzheimer's disease, had been experiencing anxiety problems and loss of hand-eye coordination, did not make adequate progress in performing the exercises. However, with him, 20-minute walks were performed, with guidance from the therapist, executing walking coordination exercises (walking backwards and forwards and zigzagging).

Although the recommended time for collecting information for a life history is approximately 6 months, in the short period of time relevant information was collected in the user's clinical history. The time was short but having worked in physiotherapy with exercises, games, circuits, was a support for the users to have confidence in talking about details of their lives; the image of the therapist was modified, he was not the professional who performed an intervention, he was a fellow resident with whom they shared a pleasant moment while they exercised and talked.

When carrying out physiotherapy with the MACP approach, the therapist-patient dialogue was modified to a dialogue of fellow residents, the hierarchy is maintained, but it is a horizontal treatment, the user has the confidence to propose changes in their treatment. As a health professional, the working vision has changed, as I know important details of people's lives, I can approach the treatment with a different, assertive and global approach, making the user, despite their dementia or depression problems, more receptive, sociable and with a positive predisposition when carrying out treatment.

The life story is marked in the memory of the professional, understanding that behind a lost look there is a person who lived experiences, was an axis for a family, marked the life of other people, was a son, uncle or a loving father, in his golden years requires medical assistance and special care. At the end of the study, one of the users passed away, for his family it was a pleasant memory to have the life story of someone so dear to them.

Below is an excerpt from each life story:

"Betty .... I thought about becoming a nun but decided to join the order when I was 40 and was told it was too late. But I always attended prayer every Sunday and Holy Hour on Thursdays with the OSCUS sisters. I love prayer and religious life, so I never thought of getting married.

"Carlos .... We always lived as a family, I liked to play alone, I picked up worms and put them in a jar with water, I talked with the ants, I played football and marbles. I loved to sing religious music with my mother and play the piano, especially the song "Ya no he de volver". I like to write poems, short stories, some of them have been published in the Casa de la Cultura ¨ La música¨ created in 1975 and ¨Musgo y Guarida¨ which was published in 1983".

"Lidia... I have several health problems; because of my left hip I cannot walk and I am moved in a wheelchair, my lungs are delicate and protect me from the cold, I can communicate little, but with my eyes I am attentive to everything that happens around me. Sometimes my gaze is lost in the horizon, I remember my life, I get nostalgic and cry".

"Lupita...I used to dress very elegantly and wear high heels, I love to dance and listen to pasillos especially Julio Jaramillo,...Despite my cognitive impairment and my knee pain, I like to paint, do handicrafts, and exercise. And when I can dance I do it with pleasure. I always remember my mother and name her all the time".

"Pedro .... I travelled to Havana and I like to talk about Comandante Che Guevara, I have a green cap with a red star that reminds me of him. I had a very strong disappointment in love that caused me a great depression and little by little I developed Alzheimer's. My life is quiet but my thoughts are criss-crossed by my thoughts. My life is quiet but my thoughts are criss-crossing in my head, and I don't remember many things".

"Ruth...I loved spending time at home, I learnt to play the piano when I was six years old, the song I loved was Lluvia de Rosas (Rain of Roses), I like classical music. My aunt Marujita Ortiz who was single pampered me and bought beautiful fabrics for my mother to make beautiful dresses for me. In retrospect my life was very beautiful, my

passion was my work and I think that caused problems with my husband".

7 Discussion

7.1. Scope of results

Despite the short period of application, improvements in muscle strength and coordination in their daily activities were evident. This experience could be carried out for a longer period of time and exported to other centres and other contexts because it can be beneficial for the quality of life of older people.

The vision, fundamentals of MACP applied to physiotherapy has given an individual approach considering the person as a unique, autonomous, integral being. In spite of the short time in which the programme was applied, a change in the attitude of the users towards the treatment was evidenced, as well as the personalisation of the therapy given to each user. The application of the ACP decalogue is an approach to change the vision in the area of health, which will achieve significant changes and a better response from the user to the treatments.

In the personal area, the application of ACP in the practice of physiotherapy modifies the approach in the evaluation of the user, in setting the treatment objectives considering the expectations, fears, hobbies and activities that are not to the user's liking, by considering the user's observations and proposing an individual treatment, the result was positive despite the short time of application. This proposal for intervention in the field of physiotherapy with a focus on MACP can serve as a start for a closer and more effective physiotherapeutic care, with the aim of optimising treatments and focusing on the person as a unique being.

The short implementation period gave positive results, but the programme would be improved if conducted over a period longer than 9 weeks as was the intervention by Bossers (2015) showed that compared to a control group with no exercise, a combination of aerobic and strength training is more effective than aerobic training alone in slowing cognitive and motor decline in patients with dementia. On the other hand, the trial by Lamb et al. (2018) showed that the exercise training programme improved physical fitness, but there were no notable improvements in other clinical outcomes.

Another interesting study was by Morris et al. (2017), which showed that aerobic exercise in early Alzheimer's disease is associated with benefits in functional capacity. Exercise-related gains in cardiorespiratory fitness were associated with improved memory performance and reduced hippocampal atrophy, suggesting that gains in cardiorespiratory fitness may be important in generating brain benefits. Asmidawati et al. (2014), meanwhile, conduct a Cochrane review and report that multicomponent group exercise, which generally includes resistance and balance training, reduced the rate of falls by 22% and the risk of falls by 17% in adults aged 60 years and older .

Guzmán et al. (2016), meanwhile, conducted a quantitative study with a quasi-experimental design, based on the comparison of the results obtained at the beginning and end of the study period, it was determined that the population group of institutionalised Older Adults with mild physical dependence and absence of cognitive impairment presented a decrease in both conditions after participating in the programme implemented. The capacity for independence was achieved after 10 months of physical-recreational activities, which was the duration of the intervention.

7.2. Limitations and proposals for improvement

Pandemic restrictions and containment by the National Emergency Operations Committee (Government of Ecuador) limited the implementation period of the proposal.

Cognitive impairment due to health situations, which generate states of anxiety and loss of coordination, is a limiting factor for the application of the programme.

The exercise programme is not strictly adhered to, due to variations in the emotional, cognitive, health and psychological state of each resident in its implementation.

As a point for improvement, it is important to train nursing staff to collaborate in the independence of each resident's activities.

7.3. Future lines

Extend this physiotherapy intervention to a comprehensive ACP-based physiotherapy programme that maintains an interdisciplinary and individual approach for each resident.

Focus on the needs of the patient, taking a global view of the disease, obtaining a complete perspective of the physical, psychological, emotional and social situation of each user. Physiotherapeutic treatments must be socialised with the user, and with an adequate criteria and explanation of the benefits, reach a consensus or change of treatment, and carry out an assertive and effective dialogue between therapist - user.

8 Conclusions

Despite the short implementation of the programme, the importance of an individualised programme for each resident was evident, in which a time schedule is drawn up, giving the importance and care that each person requires.

As it was a personalised programme, the residents were more interested in doing the exercises and felt important, loved and esteemed by the therapist.

The implementation of a therapeutic treatment taking into account the recommendations of the older adult, gives a positive and effective result to the intervention.

An interdisciplinary approach in the physiotherapy medical record allows for a global and efficient therapeutic intervention.

Including the Life History in the Resident's Logbook gives a global approach to the interdisciplinary team.

9 Bibliographical references

Asmidawati, A., Hamid, T. A., Hussain, R. M., & Hill, K. D. (2014). *Home based exercise to improve turning and mobility performance among community dwelling older adults: Protocol for a randomized controlled trial. BMC Geriatrics, 14* doi: http://dx.doi.org.universidadviu.idm.oclc.org/10.1186/1471-2318-14-100

Bernal, E., Faus, V., Bernal, R. (2006). *Presbyvertigo: vestibular exercises*. Gerokomos, *17*(4). https://scielo.isciii.es/scielo.php?script=sci_arttext&pid=S1134-928X2006000400004

Bossers, W., (2015). *A 9-Week Aerobic and Strength Training Program Improves Cognitive and Motor Function in Patients with Dementia: A Randomized, Controlled Trial.* PubMed. https://pubmed.ncbi.nlm.nih.gov/25648055/

Botero, B., and Pico, M. (2007). *Health-related quality of life (HRQoL) in adults over 60: A theoretical approach. Towards health promotion, 12,* 11-24. Retrieved from: http://www.scielo.org.co/pdf/hpsal/v12n1/v12n1a01.pdf

Bull, F. C., Al-Ansari, S. S., Biddle, S., Borodulin, K., Buman, M. P., Cardon, G., Carty, C., Chaput, J. P., Chastin, S., Chou, R., Dempsey, P. C., DiPietro, L., Ekelund, U., Firth, J., Friedenreich, C. M., Garcia, L., Gichu, M., Jago, R., Katzmarzyk, P. T., Lambert, E. and Willumsen, J. F. (2020). *World Health Organization 2020 guidelines on physical activity and sedentary behaviour. British journal of sports medicine, 54*(24), 1451-1462. https://doi.org/10.1136/bjsports-2020-102955

Capurro N, and Rada G, (2007). The diagnostic process. *Revista médica de Chile, 135*(4). https://doi.org/10.4067/s0034-98872007000400018

De la Rosa, A., Olaso-Gonzalez, G., Arc-Chagnaud, C., Millan, F., Salvador-Pascual, A., García-Lucerga, C., Blasco-Lafarga, C., Garcia-Dominguez, E., Carretero, A., Correas, A. G., Viña, J., and Gomez-Cabrera, M. C. (2020). *Physical exercise in the prevention and treatment of Alzheimer's disease. Journal of sport and health science, 9*(5), 394-404. https://doi.org/10.1016/j.jshs.2020.01.004

De las Peñas, C. F., and Ortiz, A. M., (2013). *Kinesitherapy, physiological bases and practical application* 1st Edition. Elsevier

D'Hyver, C. (2017). Comprehensive geriatric assessment. *Revista de la Facultad de Medicina de laUNAM, 60*(3) ,38-54. https://www.revistafacmed.com/index.php?option=com_phocadownload&view=file&id=902:valoracin-geritrica-integral&Itemid=79

Díaz-Veiga, P., Salazar, J., Etxaniz, N. and Matia Instituto Gerontológico (2017). *Module II: Conceptual bases of the Person-Centred Integrated Care Model from assessment to intervention. An approach to the* ACP model. Editorial International University of Valencia.

Díaz-Veiga, P., Salazar, J., Etxaniz, N., and Matia Instituto Gerontológico (2017). *Person-Centred Care in Gerontology: An approach to the ACP Model*. Editorial International University of Valencia.

El Haj, M., & Gallouj, K. (2019). *Self-defining Memories in Normal Aging. Current aging science, 12*(1), 43-48. https://doi.org/10.2174/1874609812666190429130052

García María (2013) Manual de ejercicio físico para personas de edad edad https://fiapam.org/wp-content/uploads/2013/07/manual-cast-ultima.pdf

Goudriaan, I., van Boekel, L. C., Verbiest, M., van Hoof, J., and Luijkx, K. G. (2021). *Dementia Enlightened? A Systematic Literature Review of the Influence of Indoor Environmental Light on the Health of Older Persons with Dementia in Long-Term Care Facilities. Clinical interventions in aging, 16*, 909-937. https://doi.org/10.2147/CIA.S297865

Guzmán-Olea, Eduardo, Pimentel-Pérez, Bertha Maribel, Salas-Casas, Andrés, Armenta-Carrasco, Anthony Iván, Oliver-González, Leslie Betzabeth, and Agis-Juárez, Raúl A.... (2016). *Prevention of physical dependence and cognitive impairment through the implementation of an early rehabilitation program in institutionalized older adults. Acta universitaria, 26*(6), 53-59. https://doi.org/10.15174/au.2016.1056

Hortobágyi, T., Granacher, U., Fernandez-Del-Olmo, M., Howatson, G., Manca, A., Deriu, F., Taube, W., Gruber, M., Márquez, G., Lundbye-Jensen, J., and Colomer-Poveda, D. (2021). *Functional relevance of resistance training-induced neuroplasticity in health and disease. Neuroscience and biobehavioral reviews, 122*, 79-91. https://doi.org/10.1016/j.neubiorev.2020.12.019

Howard, E. P., Schreiber, R., Morris, J. N., Russotto, A., and Flashner-Fineman, S. (2016). COLLAGE 360: *A Model of Person-Centered Care To Promote Health Among Older Adults. Journal of ageing research and healthcare, 1*(1), 21-30. https://doi.org/10.14302/issn.2474-7785.jarh-16-1123

Hsu, C. Y., Wu, H. H. H., Liao, H. E., Liao, T. H., Su, S. C., & Lin, P. S. (2021). *Self-monitored versus supervised walking programs*

for older adults. Medicine, 100(16), e25561.
https://doi.org/10.1097/MD.0000000000025561

*Official College of Physiotherapists of the Valencian Community (*2021). COLFISIOCV. https://www.colfisiocv.com

Kottke Frederic, & ,Lehmann Justus (2002). *Physical medicine and rehabilitation* (Fourth edition ed., Vol. 1). Editorial Médica Panamericana.

Kousha, A., Sayedi, A., Rezakhani, H., and Matlabi, H. (2020). The Iranian Protocol of Group Reminiscence and Health-Related Quality of Life Among Institutionalized Older People. *Journal of Multidisciplinary Healthcare, 13*, 1027-1034.
https://doi.org/10.2147/jmdh.s263421

Lamb, S. E., Sheehan, B., Atherton, N., Nichols, V., Collins, H., Mistry, D., Dosanjh, S., Slowther, A. M., Khan, I., Petrou, S., and Lall, R. (2018). *Dementia and Physical Activity (DAPA) trial of moderate to high intensity exercise training for people with dementia: randomised controlled trial. BMJ, k1675.* https://doi.org/10.1136/bmj.k1675

Lind, M., Bluck, S., and McAdams, D. P. (2021). More Vulnerable? The Life Story Approach Highlights Older People's Potential for Strength During the Pandemic. *The journals of gerontology. Series B, Psychological sciences and social sciences, 76*(2), e45-e48. https://doi.org/10.1093/geronb/gbaa105

López-Cano, M. A., Navarro, B., Nieto, M., Andrés-Pretel, F., & Latorre, J. M. (2020). *Autobiographical emotional induction in older people through popular songs: Effect of reminiscence bump and enculturation. PloS one, 15(9), e0238434.* https://doi.

Mantilla, Alfonso (2018). *Physiotherapeutic assessment instruments in adult and paediatric populations: Used in clinical practice; a review of the literature.* Journal Movimiento Scientific issn-l:2011-7191, 12 (2), 13-22 https://dialnet.unirioja.es/servlet/articulo?codigo=6985061

Martínez, T. (2013). *Person-centred care.* http://www.acpgerontologia.com.

Moreno, María José (2017) *Evaluation of environments from the Person-Centred Care Model: accessibility and environmental design* Editorial Universidad Internacional de Valencia.

Morris, J. K., Vidoni, E. D., Johnson, D. K., Van Sciver, A., Mahnken, J. D., Honea, R. A., Wilkins, H. M., Brooks, W. M., Billinger, S. A., Swerdlow, R. H., and Burns, J. M. (2017). *Aerobic exercise for Alzheimer's disease: A randomized controlled pilot trial. PLOS ONE, 12*(2), e0170547. https://doi.org/10.1371/journal.pone.0170547

World Health Organization (2006). CD47.R1 *Disability: prevention and rehabilitation in the context of the right to the enjoyment of the highest attainable standard of physical and mental health and other related rights.* https://www.paho.org/es/documentos/cd47r1-discapacidad-prevencion-rehabilitacion-contexto-derecho-al-disfrute-mas-alto accessed 23/04/2021

World Health Organization (2015, 3 October). *Good health adds life to years.* https://apps.who.int/iris/handle/10665/75254

World Health Organization. (2017). *10 facts about ageing and health.* https://www.who.int/es/news-room/fact-sheets/detail/envejecimiento-y-salud

United Nations Educational, Scientific and Cultural Organization (2018). Social responsibility and health. Report of the International Bioethics Committee of UNESCO. Logroño. http://www.cibir.es/files/biblioteca/2018-UNESCO-Bioetica.pdf

Romero, L. (2016, 2 August). *Frenkel exercises*. E Fisioterapia. https://www.efisioterapia.net/articulos/ejercicios-frenkel

Unutmaz, G. D., Soysal, P., Tuven, B., & Isik, A. T. (2018*). Costs of medication in older patients: before and after comprehensive geriatric assessment. Clinical interventions in aging, 13*, 607-613. https://doi.org/10.2147/CIA.S159966

Yanguas, J., and Sánchez J. A. (2017). *Strategic and operational planning according to the ACP Model: Project and process design.* Editorial Universidad Internacional de Valencia.

10. Annexes

Annex 1. User data collection

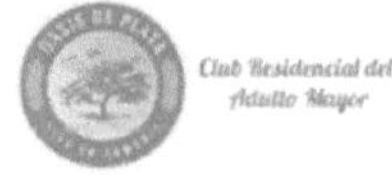

Quito, 21 de abril de 2021

Señores
Universidad Internacional de Valencia
Quito

De mi consideración:

Por medio del presente Oasis de Plata Club Residencial del Adulto Mayor, centro gerontológico, autoriza a la señora Lic. Raquel Elizabeth Rivera Vargas, a recoger la información necesaria sobre los expedientes de los usuarios para elaborar su Trabajo de Final del Máster Universitario en Gerontología y Atención centrada en la persona de la Universidad Internacional de Valencia.

La información que recoja deberá mantenerse en reserva y será utilizada únicamente para el trabajo final.

Atentamente,

Sharon Herrera Camacho
DIRECTORA DE OASIS DE PLATA

CC. Lic. Raquel Rivera

Annex 2. Informed Consent

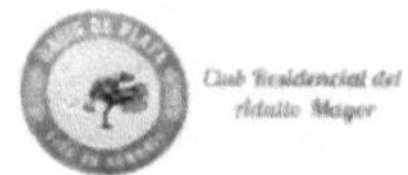

Quito, 22 de Abril del 2021

CONSENTIMIENTO INFORMADO

Yo, con C.C epresentante legal de con C.C. residente del Club Residencial del Adulto Mayor Oasis de La Plata, centro gerόntológico autorizo para que a mi representado se le realice una valoración fisioterapéutica y crear una historia de vida.

Valoración que la realizará la Lic. Raquel Elizabeth Rivera Vargas, Fisioterapeuta, alumna del Máster de Gerontología y Atención Centrada en la Persona de la Universidad Internacional de Valencia.

Atentamente,

C.C

Annex 3 Physiotherapy Medical Records

HISTORIA CLINICA FISIOTERAPEUTICA

FECHA RECOLECCION DE DATOS:

NOMBRE: C.C.

EDAD: Fecha Nacimiento

ESTADO CIVIL: PROFESION:

DIAGNOSTICO:

RECOMENDACIONES EQUIPO INTERDICIPLINARIO

MEDICO GERIATRA

PSICOLOGA

PSIQUIATRA

TRABAJADORA SOCIAL

TERAPEUTA OCUPACIONAL

PROFESOR DE EDUCACION FISICA

MEDICACIÓN

pág. 1

HISTORIA CLINICA FISIOTERAPEUTICA

ANTECEDENTES RELEVANTES DE SU HISTORIA DE VIDA (lo que le gusta y no le gusta a la persona)

ANTECEDENTES CLINICOS

EXAMEN FÍSICO

TEST POSTURAL

TEST DE DANIELS

ESCALA TINETTI

ESCALA DE BERG

PRUEBA DE BALANCE

PRUEBA DE VELOCIDAD AL CAMINAR

PRUEVA DE LEVANTARSE DE LA SILLA

ESCALA ROSOW-BRESLAU

MOVILIDAD ARTICULAR

ARTICULACION	DERECHO	IZQUIERDO
HOMBRO		
CODO		
MUÑECA		
DEDOS		
CADERA		
RODILLA		
TOBILLOS		
DEDOS		
COLUMNA		

pág. 2

HISTORIA CLINICA FISIOTERAPEUTICA

PLAN DE TRATAMIENTO FISIOTERAPEUTICO

Objetivo

Tiempo de tratamiento

Descripción tratamiento

Observaciones y Recomendaciones

Firma del Fisioterapeuta

pág. 3

ANNEX MODEL LIFE HISTORY

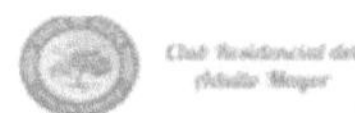

Historia de Vida

De……………

FOTO

Soy, nací en Quito el 20 de Abril de….., viví con mi madre …., mi abuelita Rosa y mi hermano mayor Gerardo, mi madre murió cuando tenía 13 años con cáncer de mama.

Estudié en un internado de la Providencia. Me gradué de secretaria bilingüe y trabajé en Andinatel, cuando fui mayor de edad viví en una residencia donde por medio de una amiga española conocí a las hermanas religiosas de Obra Social Cultural Sopeña (OSCUS), me encariñé mucho con ellas a los 30 años fui a trabajar a España en una agencia de turismo en Madrid durante 4 años, regresé a Ecuador porque tenía episodios de ausencias.

Mi hermano actualmente está divorciado pero tiene 4 hijos, Paulina, Esteban, Javier y Paty. Con los que tengo comunicación son Paulina y Esteban que están pendientes de mí.

Pensé en hacerme religiosa pero me decidí en ingresar a la orden cuando tenía 40 años y me dijeron que era muy tarde. Pero siempre asistía todos los domingos a la oración y a la hora santa los jueves con las hermanas de OSCUS. También asistí a los talleres de Manualidades y Primeros auxilios.

En OSCUS tenía una hermana religiosa Patrocinio de cariño le decían Patzi, yo la quería mucho y la llamaba mamá, murió hace un año.

Me gusta mucho rezar, y la vida religiosa por eso nunca pensé en casarme.

El señor dio su vida por los pecadores, se entregó

Siempre pensé estar en una residencia de mayores, cuando me enseño en una parte ya no quiero salir.

Mis diagnósticos son epilepsia con periodos de ausencias, uso audífono izquierdo, para trasladarme ando con bastón con medio de precaución para no caerme.

Me siento tranquila, estoy enseñada aquí, me gusta el pollo frito, leer el periódico y ver las noticias para estar informada.

………. fallece el 1 de Junio de 2021

"Padre nuestro tu que estás en los que aman la verdad,
Has que el Reino que por ti se dio llegue pronto a nuestro corazón,
Que el amor, que tu hijo, nos dejó, ese amor, reine ya… en nosotros,
Y en el pan de la unidad Cristo danos tú la paz,
Y olvídate de nuestro mal,
si olvidamos el de los demás,
no permitas, que caigamos en tentación…
Oh Señor, y ten piedad del mundo… "

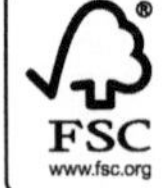

MIX
Papier aus verantwortungsvollen Quellen
Paper from responsible sources
FSC® C105338

Printed by Books on Demand GmbH, Norderstedt / Germany